Improving Productivity in the Workplace: A Do-It-Yourselfer's Guide to Being More Productive, Efficient, and Happy

By Dr. Carey Heller

Introduction

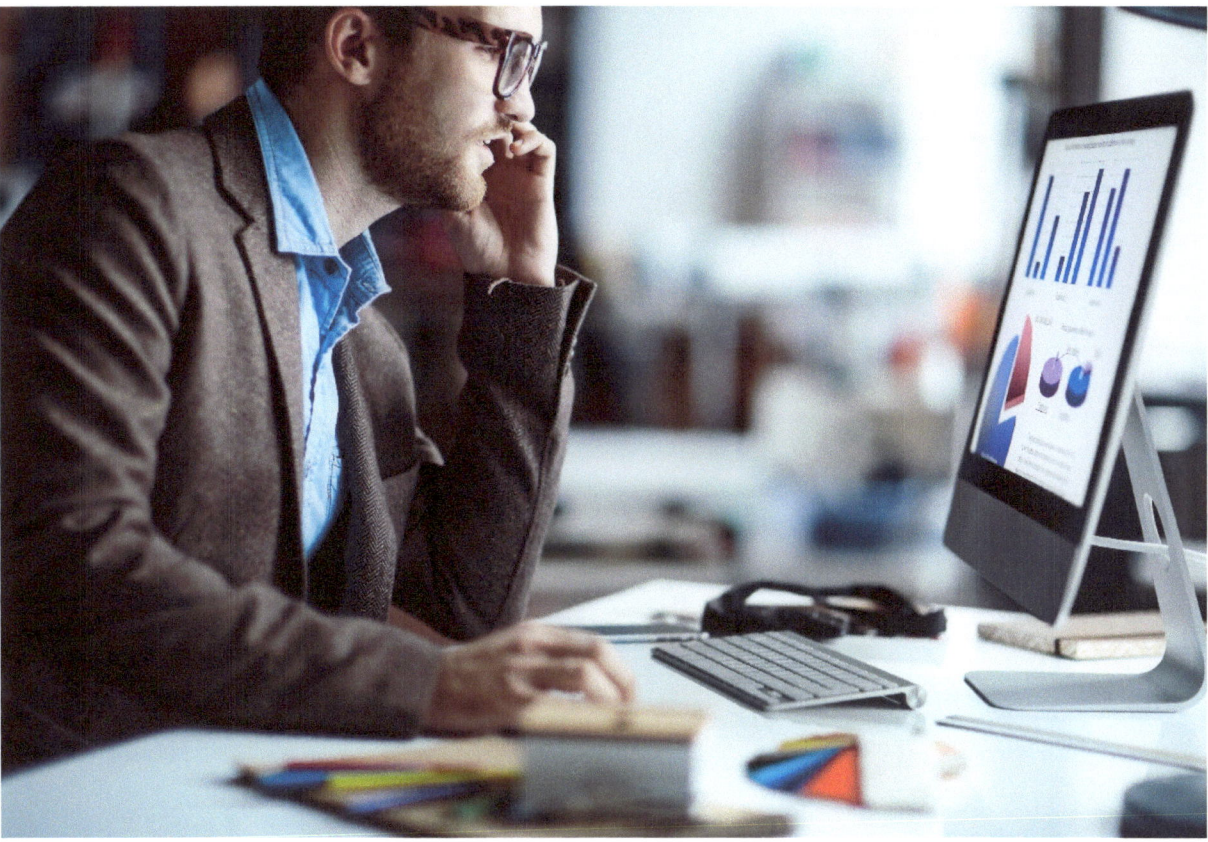

- Do you wish there were more hours in the day to get things done?
- Are you frequently falling behind on tasks at work?
- Do you feel that you would be much more productive if you didn't have to check email or make phone calls as often?
- Do you feel like you work all the time?
- Do you wish you could enjoy life outside of work more?

If the answer to any of these questions is "yes," you've picked the right book to read. While this book could certainly be several hundred pages detailing every way you can make improvements to increase your productivity, which in turn may improve your happiness and life satisfaction, reading such a long book wouldn't be an efficient use of your time. Thus, this book contains a variety of questions to get you thinking about how you approach different aspects of your job. In addition, practical tools to help you make changes are discussed. It is crucial to keep in mind that everybody functions differently, even in the same job, so tools need to be tailored to meet your individual needs. While it is difficult to encompass all types of jobs in a productivity book, this book is geared towards professions that involve a lot of time in an office. Nonetheless, it is the principles included in this book that I hope will be most helpful in allowing you to make changes to help yourself, and these principles transcend most professions.

NOTES

Chapter 1: The Basics of Task Management

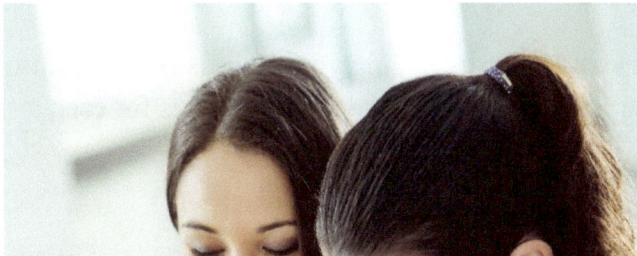

Unless you have a job that involves doing the same thing over and over again (i.e., adding a part to an item on an assembly line), chances are you have a variety of tasks that you need to complete as part of your job. Knowing what tasks you need to complete is crucial in not only completing them, but figuring out how to do so most efficiently.

Exercise:

1. *Write or type out all tasks that you have to complete.*
2. *Pick three or four categories in which tasks can be classified based on frequency or type (i.e, one time, daily, marketing).*
3. *Put items from your list under the proper category.*

What you have done right here is figure out everything that you have to do. In addition, by categorizing it, it breaks down the number of tasks into more manageable numbers by category so you can better organize yourself. If you have 30 tasks in one list, while they all might be there, chances are it may be overwhelming to look at and you might miss items when going through your list of what to complete.

Exercise (Part 2): The next step in organizing your tasks is figuring out when you are going to complete them. Think about and write out the following items for each task on your list:

- *How long will it take to complete?*
- *What is the deadline to complete it by?*
- *Are there certain times of day in which it has to be completed? (i.e., before 10 AM)*
- *Is there travel time involved?*
- *If it is a big task (i.e, planning an event), what parts can I break it into? For example:*
    - *Reserve venue*
    - *Create marketing materials*
    - *Advertise event*
    - *Reserve caterer*
    - *Hire security*

NOTES

Chapter 2: Thinking About Setting Up Your Schedule and Making a Plan to Complete Tasks

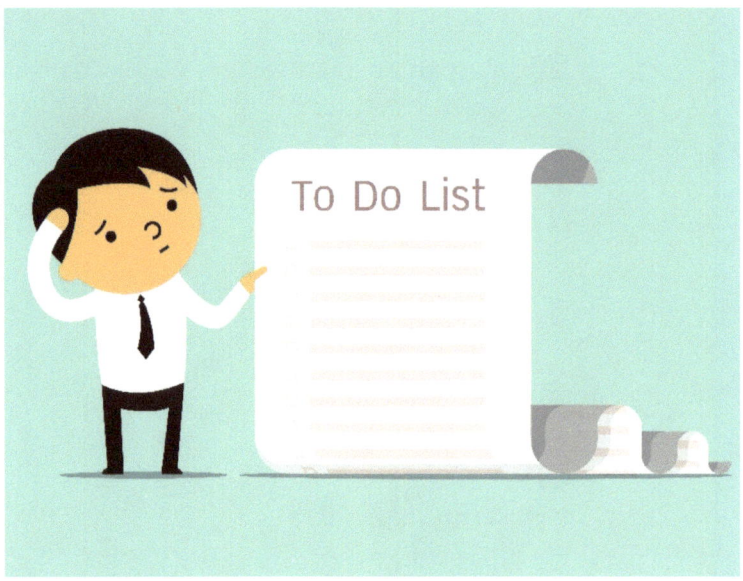

These are some things to think about before looking at revamping your schedule and making a new plan for completing tasks:

1. Do I work better with large blocks of time (i.e., three hours) or shorter chunks (i.e., 30 minutes)?
2. If I have a job that involves going out of the office a lot or always traveling to meet with clients, am I efficient with how I schedule items?
    a. For example, do you try to schedule appointments in the same small geographic area at a time or are you running across the area constantly wasting valuable time?
    b. If you do have to be on the go a lot, are you maximizing time between appointments to complete tasks (i.e., return phone calls, emails, work on projects sitting somewhere)?
3. If I have control over the scheduling of meetings in the office do I pay attention to when in the day and week they are scheduled?
    a. I.e., do you schedule too many meetings in one day that reduces your time to complete work, return emails/phone calls, etc.?
    b. I.e., do you schedule too many meetings/appointments at random times throughout the week that it doesn't leave sufficient blocks of time to complete tasks?
4. Think about how easily you can shift between tasks. I.e., does it take a long time to get started or restarted after an interruption?
5. Do you check your email constantly?
6. Do you always answer the phone if you are available or return calls as soon as you get the voicemail?

7. Are there items that I can automate more (i.e., processing payments)?

Just thinking about these items, I can imagine that you might be already starting to think about how you can make some changes in your schedule. Focus first on adjusting your face-to-face commitments. After you do so, you can really start focusing on how to be more efficient with completing items from your task list.

NOTES

Chapter 3: Suggestions for Organizational Systems

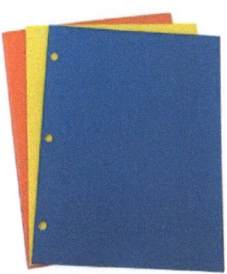

Do I want an electronic, paper, or a hybrid system?

A few points to keep in mind for electronic systems:

- Records of tasks are more portable and you are less likely to lose them
- More potential for overlooking or accidentally deleting items
- Not visible unless you are on your electronic device
- Benefit of notification reminders

A few points about paper systems:

- More visible when looking at it
- Less distractions when viewing it than on an electronic device
- More problematic if you lose list
- Less collaboration options with others (i.e., can't automatically update a shared task list)

Here are some suggestions for using an electronic system to keep track of your appointments and tasks:

1. Use an electronic calendar, preferably one that syncs with your computer, phone, tablet, etc.
   a. Put all appointments in it.
2. Use a task list app, preferably one that allows you to create multiple lists. In addition, one that syncs with your calendar may be most helpful.
   a. Some apps that connect a calendar and task list such as iCalendar, show you your task on the calendar at the designated time, which can be helpful in visualizing your whole schedule (including tasks that need to be completed). However, if you need more time blocked out than the task settings will allow, it may be better to reserve the amount of time needed in the calendar as an event.
3. Here are some suggested apps/programs:
   a. Reminders app: allows multiple lists, syncs with many third party task list apps.
   b. gTasks: syncs with Reminders app and Google Calendar/iCloud calendars.

c. Wunderlist: no calendar syncing feature, but allows you to create check boxes for subtasks.
d. Do!: Simple task list app. No calendar connected.
e. To-Do: Another simple task list app. No calendar associated with it.
f. iCalendar app: syncs with phone calendar, Google Calendar, and Reminders app.
g. Calendars app: syncs with phone calendar, Google Calendar, and Reminders app.

Here are some suggestions for using a paper organizational system:

1. Use a large paper calendar on your wall.
2. Have a small calendar that you carry with you.
3. Make sure calendars are updated daily to be the same.
4. Have paper lists of tasks, organized by category or time frequency (i.e., daily, weekly), and check off tasks when done.
   a. For reoccurring lists, make a copy and write in the date each time you change the list so you do not have to rewrite it constantly.
5. Consider scanning your lists daily or as needed to a cloud system such as Google Drive or Dropbox to back them up and have access to them remotely. You can take a picture of the lists on your phone, and upload them to your cloud account instantly.
6. Use a whiteboard to keep track of tasks or for a daily to-do list.

Regardless of whether you use an electronic, paper, or hybrid system, here are some key components of a successful organizational plan:

1. Make a daily to-do list from your master to-do lists
   a. This avoids wasting time figuring out what to do during the day.
2. List out the estimated completion time of each task and schedule it on your calendar or task list at a time when you anticipate being able to complete it.
3. If tasks do not get completed when scheduled, reschedule them for another time.
4. Block out specific periods of time to complete important tasks and treat these as an appointment by not scheduling anything during these times.
5. Reserve time in your schedule to catch up or get ahead on items, especially times on Mondays and Fridays, to make weekend transitions easier.

NOTES

Chapter 4: Examples of Organizational Systems

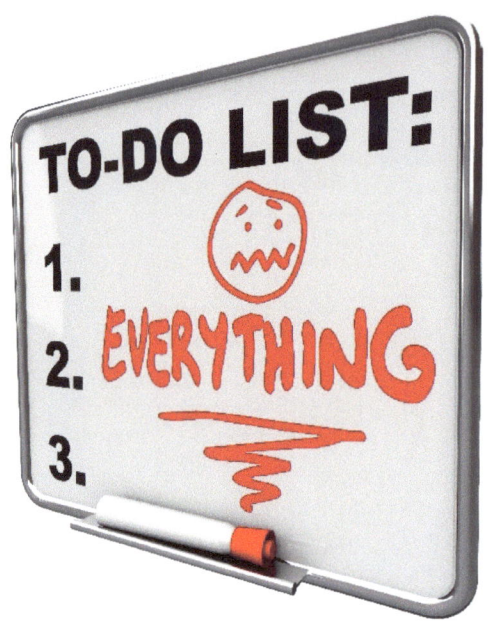

Sample Task List Organized by Reoccurrence Frequency (Could be used electronically in app or on paper):

Reoccurring Weekly

Item	When to Complete It	Estimated Completion Time
Submit information to payroll company	Friday at 10 AM	1 hour
Inventory	Monday at 9 AM	2 hours
Check online marketing	Wednesday at 4 PM	15 minutes
Update computer software	Thursday at 10 AM	2 hours
Reconcile transactions	Friday at 4 PM	20 minutes

Reoccurring Monthly

Item	When to Complete It	Estimated Completion Time
Pay credit card bill	Monday the 24th at 10 AM	10 minutes
Update monthly orders for supplies	Thursday the 1st at 8 AM	1 hour
Update website	Wednesday the 10th at 2 PM	20 minutes
Send final notices to clients who have not paid	Thursday the 1st at 9 AM	1 hour

One-Time

Item	When to Complete It	Estimated Completion Time
Pay plumber bill	Tuesday at 10 AM	10 minutes
Plan networking event Find venue Select food Get speaker Create marketing tools Market event	Monday at 2 PM	Unknown
Buy new computer	Wednesday at 4 PM	1 hour
Update insurance	Tuesday at 4 PM	15 minutes

Sample Task List Organized by Category (Could be used electronically in app or on paper):

Marketing

Item	When to Complete It	Estimated Completion Time
Design new brochures	Tuesday at 9 AM	2 hours
Get brochures printed	Tuesday at 1 PM	10 minutes
Update website	Wednesday at 12 PM	30 minutes
Order pens	Tuesday at 10 AM	20 minutes

Projects

Item	When to Work on It Next	Estimated Completion Time
Proposal for gym	Tuesday from 2 PM to 4 PM	2 hours
Article for journal	Monday at 3 PM	1 hour
Analysis for garden	Thursday at 10 AM	2 hours

Contact Tasks

Item	When to Complete	Method of Contact/If Need to Follow Up
Jack Jameson about scheduling meeting	Wednesday at 1 PM	Email: follow up if no response in one day
Joel Book about outstanding payment	Tuesday at 3 PM	Call: follow up with letter if no response within two days

Sample Electronic System:

Sample 1:

- iCalendar app synced with smartphone using Google Calendar for appointments and to block out time to complete tasks.
- Reminders app also synced with iCalendar to keep track of tasks based on frequency and category, which show up in list form and on the calendar at the time they are scheduled to be completed.

Sample 2:

- Microsoft Outlook Calendar synced with smartphone for appointments.
- Wunderlist app for tasks.

Sample 3:

- Microsoft Outlook Calendar synced with smartphone for appointments.
- Franklin Covey Planner integrated into Outlook to manage tasks.

Sample Paper System

Sample 1:

- All tasks listed by category written on giant white board. In the middle, the tasks that are intended to be completed today are written.
- Take picture of white board at the end of each day for records.
- Paper calendar to keep track of appointments.

Sample 2:

- Piece of paper with all tasks listed out.
- Daily to-do list written with time scheduled to complete each task during the day.
- Large wall calendar as well as portable paper calendar to keep track of appointments.
  - Use the portable calendar as the primary one, and update the wall calendar at the end of each day.

Sample 3:

- Master to-do list on piece of paper organized by category.
- Each item that needs to be completed today is copied onto a sticky note and the sticky note is put into the completed pile once the task is complete.
- Paper calendar to keep track of appointments.

Sample Hybrid Paper/Electronic System

Sample 1:

- Use calendar app that comes standard with phone synced with email address to keep track of appointments and block out time to complete tasks.
- Master task list kept on Do! app.
- Daily to-do list written out by hand.

Sample 2:

- Use paper calendar to manage appointments and block out time to complete tasks.
- Wunderlist app to keep track of tasks.

Sample 3:

- Use Google Calendar (synced between computer and phone) to keep track of appointments and block out time as needed.
- Paper master to-do list.
- Daily to-do list written out by hand.

NOTES

Chapter 5: A Few Points on Office Efficiency

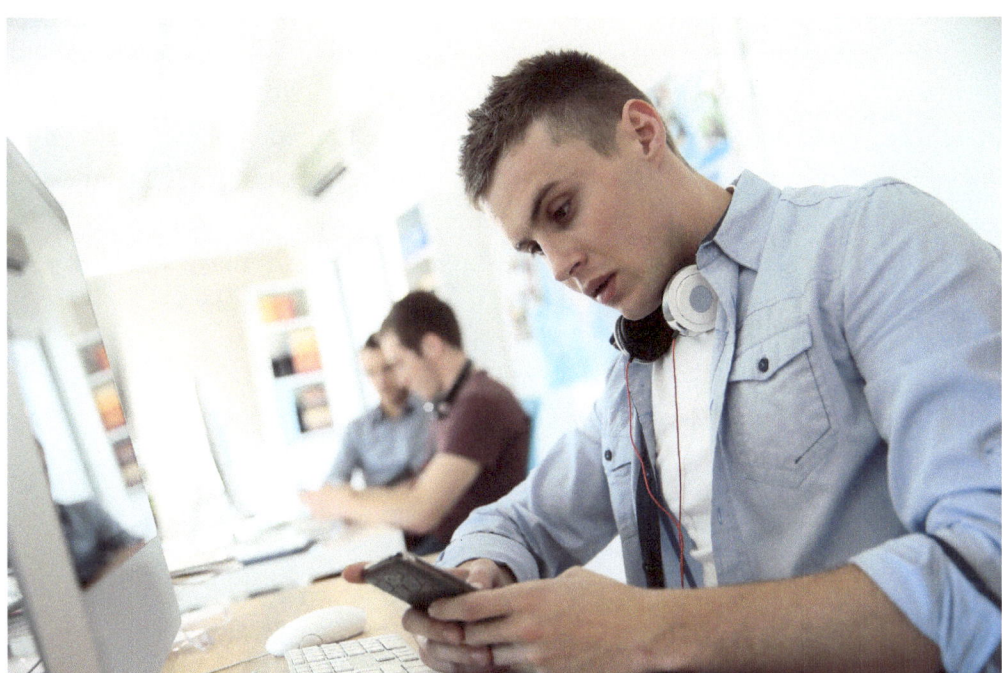

Communication with others, whether via email, phone, text, or in person is often a vital element of a job. At the same time, these can also be a major impediment to being productive if not scheduled properly.

Email:

- Unless you have a job that requires you to respond instantaneously to email, consider checking your email a set intervals throughout the day and blocking out time to respond rather than responding each time you get one.
  - You lose valuable time each time you stop to check and respond to an email and then likely need additional time to regain focus on whatever task you were completing.
  - Depending on your field, some clients send many emails a day, and if you wait before responding, individuals tend to combine their needs into fewer emails or may even be more likely to wait until they meet with you next to ask rather than continuing to send you many emails a day. This also avoids getting into back and forth conversations via email.

Phone:

- If you don't have a job that requires you to constantly answer your phone, consider letting it go to voicemail all the time, or at least when you are busy working on a task. Maybe even turn the ringer off. Not answering your phone while you are busy will increase your productivity because you aren't shifting your attention from a task to a phone call, and then back again. Reserve time in your schedule multiple times a day to check and respond to voicemails, or if feasible, set aside a call hour or two where people know they can call during set times and you will pick up. Not answering all calls directly also allows you to get projects completed and devote time to phone calls on your schedule. In some environments, you may not even be the right person to speak with, and you can forward the contact information onto the correct person without having to take the time to speak with the person in the first place. Of course, make sure that your company allows you to not answer the phone if you are at your desk.

NOTES

Chapter 6: Reducing Distractions

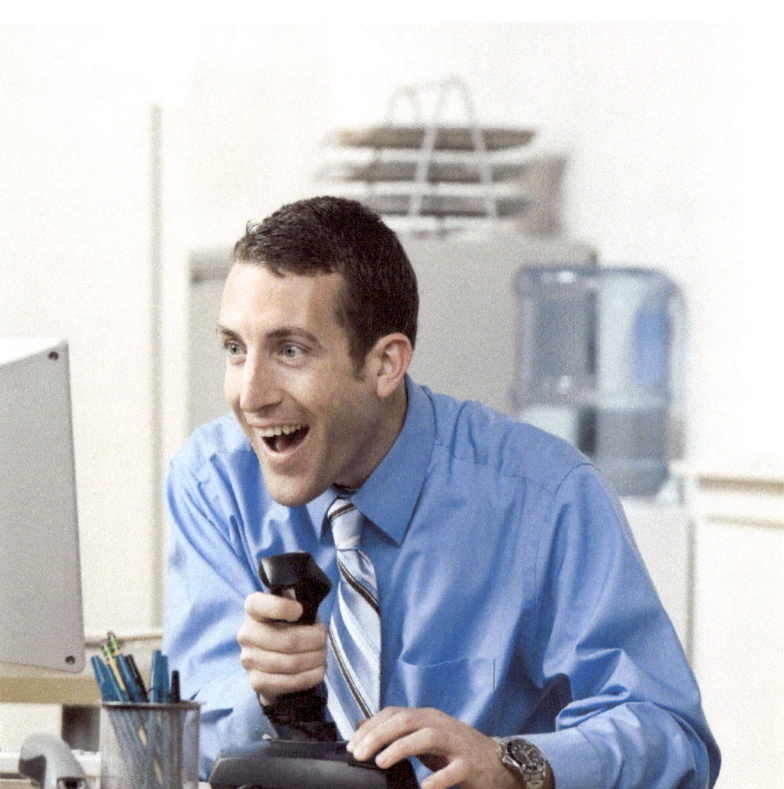

Cell Phone:

- Unless you are using your phone for work, put it on silent, and set it so only important alerts come through.

Internet:

- Don't keep non-work websites open. However, if you feel that you need to do so, ideally create a separate user profile and only access websites for personal use during breaks (and use a timer to avoid spending too much time during your break), use a different web browser for personal sites, or use web browser extensions to block access to sites that would distract you except during set break times. Of course, if your company does not allow you to access personal websites, that may make it a bit easier to not be tempted to access them during work hours.

NOTES

Chapter 7: Improving Focus

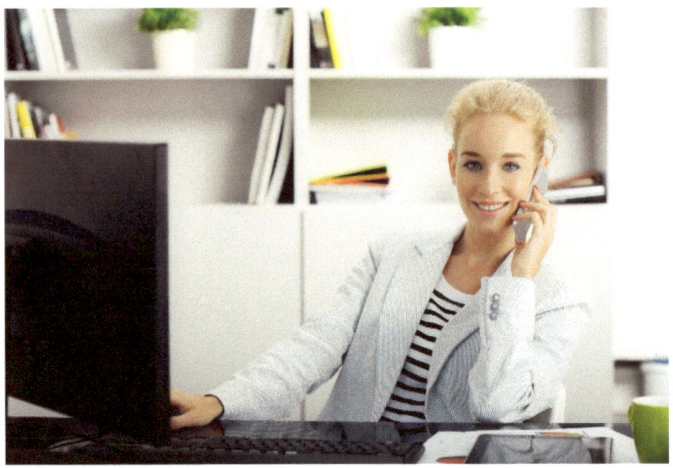

Organizational system: Having a good organizational system will likely keep you better focused and on task.

Workspace: Making sure your desk is clear of items unless you need them regularly can be useful. Also making sure that you have items that you use frequently within arms reach of your desk reduces the frequency of which you have to get up and find specific items. Less items around your workspace also leads to less distractions and better focus.

Interval Apps: For some individuals it is especially difficult to remain focused. Using interval apps such as Seconds allows one to have chimes or vibrations go off at set intervals, which jolt you if you've zoned out and over time individuals associate the chimes/vibrations with reminders to stay on task.

Physical activity: Regular physical activity is important for a variety of reasons. Being healthier in of itself can improve productivity and many people find that working out before work helps them be better focused throughout the day.

Tools to minimize fidgeting: Some individuals struggle to sit for long periods of time and get restless and/or fidget. If you fall into this category, try something physical while you are working such as using a small bicycle or elliptical machine under your desk, exercise bands on your chair, tennis balls cut in half and taped to the floor, or other items that would provide you with simple movement. The goal is to find something that occupies your feet without being distracting. Many people find that harnessing fidgeting can lead to greater focus.

Take breaks: Pick set times of the day to have breaks and plan out ahead of time what you will do for the break and how long you will take. This gives you something to look forward to and makes it easier to get back on task after a break since the time is preset. In addition, people are often more refreshed after a break and will likely be more productive than if they had sat doing the same task for hours on end without a break.

NOTES

Chapter 8: Running Your Own Business

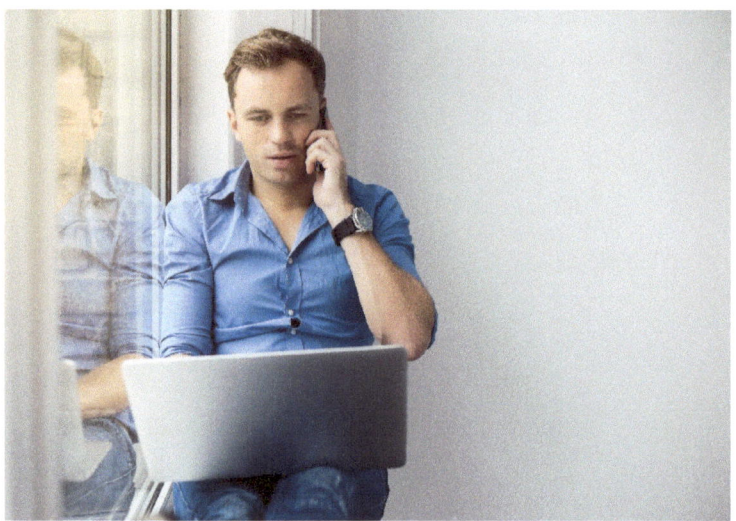

If you run your own business, many of the tools discussed above will be relevant. In addition, you have the benefit of presumably having more control over your work hours, environment, etc. Unfortunately, that also means you probably have a lot of responsibility and possibly more tasks to do than is realistic for one person to do unless you can delegate sufficiently. Here are a few tips to keep in mind when running your own business:

1. Being efficient with time is extremely crucial.
2. Try to automate as much as you can in terms of paying bills, collecting payments, etc. to reduce time you have to devote to it.
3. Minimize how much time you spend on the phone or returning emails when possible, especially when it is not billable and it is unlikely your time spent will result in a new client or other direct benefit.
4. Evaluate your organizational system monthly and revamp it as needed.
5. Reserve time to complete different components of your job, especially ones that are often not as important in the moment, but necessary in general (i.e., marketing, updating website, etc.).

NOTES

Chapter 9: Self-Care

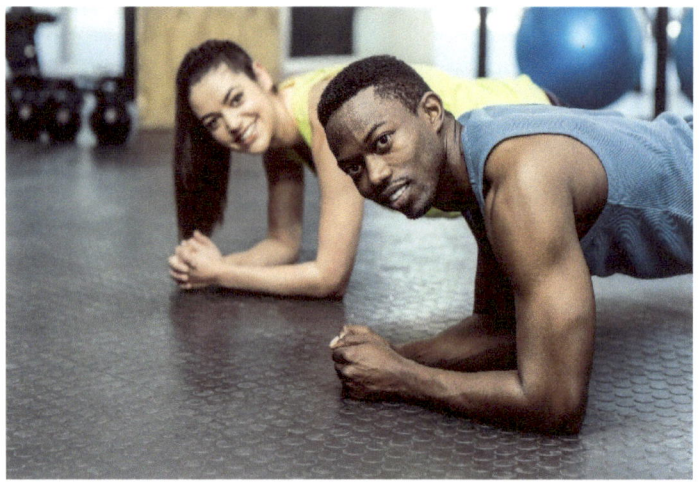

If you do not take good care of yourself, you will suffer as well as your job performance. In addition, the happier you are in general, the more efficient you likely will be. Therefore, getting enough sleep, regular exercise (also discussed above), and eating healthy are important. Taking care of your mental health is also crucial. If you are anxious, depressed, or otherwise experiencing negative feelings, you are more likely to be distracted, your cognitive functioning may be impaired, and you will be less productive. Thus, address any environmental stressors that you have control over, use mindfulness, guided visual imagery, meditation, or seek professional assistance to address any mental health issues. Furthermore, consider talking to someone at your company about employee health initiatives and/or with permission, perhaps start a weekly walk or stretch activity with co-workers.

NOTES

Chapter 10: Putting it All Together

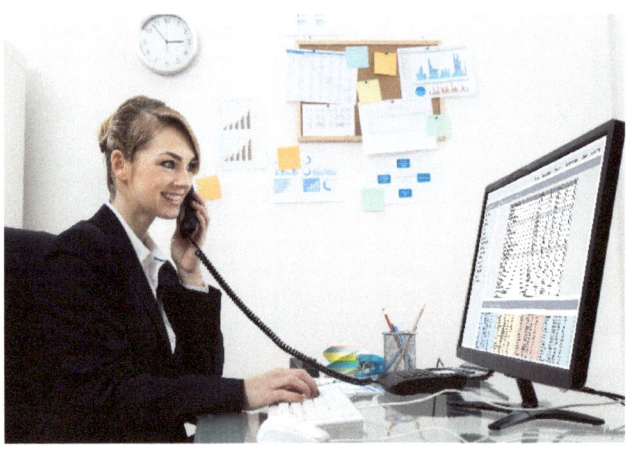

Now that you have either read or skimmed this book, you likely have viewed enough questions to get yourself thinking about how you can make changes to improve your productivity. Hopefully some of the practical suggestions will be useful as well.

No two people are the same in terms of how they work best, which is why it is important to focus on how you work and build an organizational system around that rather than simply pulling tools from random resources and trying to implement them. While pulling tools from resources such as this book can be helpful, it is more important to focus on the process of what you are doing to make changes, because that will enable you to develop skills that are more adaptable to changing demands to meet them with success.

It's great to take these ideas and tools and try to implement them on your own. For many individuals that is sufficient. However, for others, they do best with professional assistance in the form of a mental health professional or organizational coach. Such an individual will meet you where you are and hopefully work collaboratively with you to develop an organizational system that you are comfortable with and will work well. Furthermore, sometimes speaking with a supervisor about obtaining extra guidance or specific items that are small through the company (i.e., larger wall calendar) that could help you be more productive can be helpful.

NOTES

About the Author

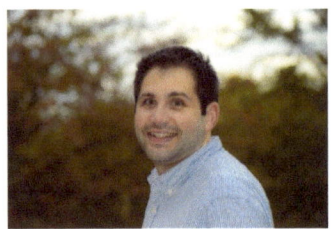

Carey Heller, Psy.D. is a clinical psychologist and founding partner of The Heller Psychology Group in Bethesda, Maryland. He specializes in evaluating and treating ADHD and executive functioning difficulties. Time management and organizational abilities are at the core of these issues. Thus, many children and teens with difficulties in these domains struggle to adapt to adulthood as well as the workforce without assistance. Dr. Heller assists individuals in improving their ability to function not only successfully, but efficiently, in childhood, adolescence, and adulthood.

For additional resources, including articles that Dr. Heller has written, please visit www.hellerpsychologygroup.com and/or follow him on Facebook and Twitter.